KETO AIR FRYER COOKBOOK

52 Quick, Easy, and Delicious Reasons Why You Will Never Have To Eat Excessively Oily Fried Food Again.

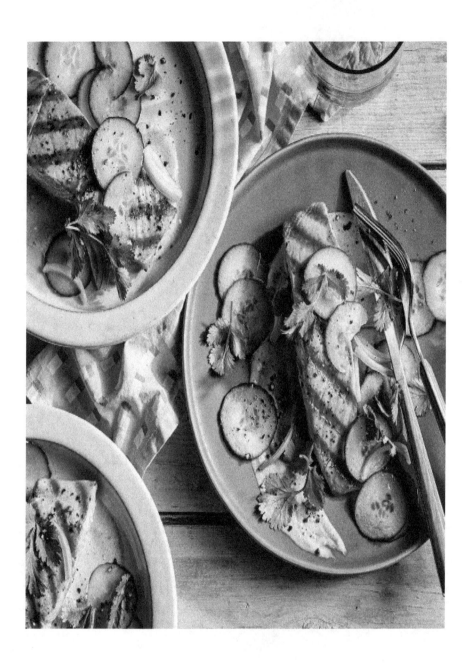

Table of Contents

Introduction

Cooking with a fryer is as easy as using a microwave. Anyone can do this, and after only a few uses, you have moved on to this amazing way of cooking before. You will be introduced to the air bowl options and maximize your cooking and creaking time, explain how to keep your adult air sweetener clean and recommend some accessories that make the frying experience even easier and more enjoyable. Although this chapter covers the basics of using an air fryer, the first step is to read the manual that has been reached to the fryer. All fryers are different, and with the recent increase in the popularity of the device, there are many different models on the market. Learning how to use a specific air fryer is the key to success and will familiarize you with troubleshooting and safety features. If you read the manual and wash all rooms with hot soapy water before first use, you'll feel ready to let go of the culinary finesse!

Why fry the air?

Frying the air is becoming increasingly popular, as it allows you to prepare delicious meals quickly and evenly with little oil and little effort. Here are some of the reasons you want to switch to frying:

Replace other kitchens. You can use the adult air sweetener in the oven, microwave oven, fryer and

Dehydrator! You can quickly prepare the perfect dishes for any meal on a small device without compromising on taste.

It cooks faster than traditional cooking methods. Air bowls work by circling hot air around the cooking chamber. The result is fast and even cook, using a fraction of the energy in the oven. Most air fryers can be adjusted to a maximum temperature of 400 degrees Celsius. It allows you to do almost everything you do in the range in the fryer.

Consume little or no cooking oil. An important selling point for air fryers is that you get beautifully cooked dishes with little or no cooking oil. While this can appeal to some because it may mean lower fat content, people who follow a keto diet can enjoy it because it means fewer calories, which is always essential if you're making keto for weight loss.

There's a quick cleaning. With all cooking methods, you are sure to get a dirty oven, but with the smallest bakery and removable air fryer basket, the complete cleaning is a bread crumb!

Cleaning the air fryer

Make sure the fryer is completely cold and off before cleaning. To clean the air, you need it:

- Remove the air from the base. And fill the bowl with hot water and washing liquid. Soak the pan for 10 minutes with a frying basket in it.
- Then thoroughly clean the basket with a sponge or brush.
- Remove the fryer's basket and wipe the lower and outer walls.
- Peel the pan with a sponge or brush.
- Let it dry and get back to the bottom of the fryer.
- To clean the outer part of the fryer, wipe the outside with a damp cloth. Next, make sure all the pieces are in the right place before embarking on the next cooking adventure.

52 Keto Air fryer Recipes

Breakfast

1. Crunchy Granola

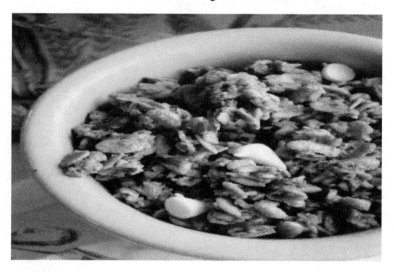

(Hands On Time: 10 minutes| Cook Time: 5 mins | Servings 6)

Things We Need

- Two mugs, pecans, chopped
- One mug unsweetened coconut flakes one mug almond slivers
- 1/3 mug sunflower seeds
- 1/4 mug golden flaxseed

- 1/4 mug low-carb, sugar-free chocolate chips
- 1/4 mug granular erythritol
- 2 tbsp. unsalted butter
- 1 tsp. ground cinnamon

Directions

In a large pan, combine all ingredients. Put the batter into a 4-mug round baking dish. Put the plate into the fryer basket. Set the temperature to 320°F and timer for 5 mins. Allow cooling completely before serving.

Nutritional Value per Serving

- Calories: 617
- Protein: 10.9grams
- Fiber: 12grams
- Net Carbohydrates:6.5grams
- sugar alcohol: 14.7grams
- Fat: 55.8grams
- Sodium: 5 mg
- Carbohydrates: 32.4grams

- sugar: 2.7grams

2. Jalapeño Popper Egg mugs

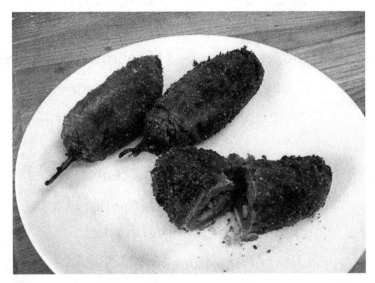

(Hands On Time: 10 minutes| Cook Time: 10 mins | Servings 1)

Things We Need

- Four large eggs

- 1/4 mug chopped pickled jalapeños

- 2 ounces full-Fat cream cheese

- 1/2 cup shredded sharp Cheddar cheese.

Directions

1. In a medium pan, beat the eggs, and then put them into four silicone muffin mugs.
2. In a large microwave-safe pan, put jalapeños, cream cheese, and Cheddar. Microwave for 30 seconds and stir. Take a spoonful, approximately 1/4
3. Of the batter, and put it in the center of one of the egg mugs. Repeat with the remaining batter.
4. Place egg mugs into the fryer basket.
5. To raise the temperature to 320°F and set the timer for 10 mins.
   Serve warm.

Nutritional Value

- Calories: 354
- Protein: 20gramsFiber: 0.2grams
- Net Carbohydrates : 2.1grams
- Fat: 25.3grams
- Sodium: 601 mg
- Carbohydrates: 2.3grams
- sugar: 4grams

3. Crispy Southwestern Ham Egg mugs

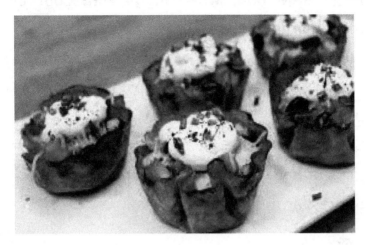

Serving 2

(Hands On Time: 5 minutes| Cook Time: 12 mins | Servings 1)

Things We Need

- 4 (1-ounce) slices of deli ham four large eggs
- 2 tbsp. full-Fat sour cream 1/4 mug diced green bell pepper 2 tbsp. chopped red bell pepper 2 tbsp. chopped white onion 1/2 mug shredded medium Cheddar cheese

Directions

1. Put one slice of ham on the bottom of four baking mugs.

2. In a large pan, whisk eggs with sour cream: mixing green pepper, red pepper, and onion.
3. Put the egg batter into ham-lined baking mugs. Top with Cheddar. Put cups into the air fryer basket.
4. Set the temperature to 320°F and timer for 12 mins or until the tops are browned.
5. Serve warm.

Nutritional Value

- Calories: 382
- Protein: 29.4grams
- Fiber: 4grams
- Net Carbohydrates : 4.6grams
- Fat: 23.6grams
- Sodium: 977 mg
- Carbohydrates: 6.0gramssugar: 2.1grams

4.   Buffalo Egg mugs

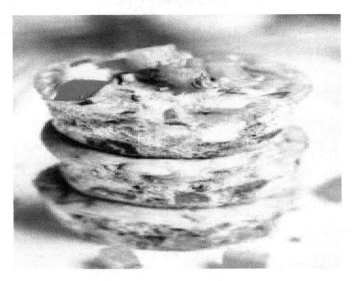

Serving 3

(Hands On Time: 10 minutes| Cook Time: 15 mins | Servings 1)

Things We Need

- Four large eggs
- 2 ounces full-Fat cream cheese
- 2 tbsp. buffalo sauce
- 1/2 mug shredded sharp Cheddar cheese

Directions

1. Crack eggs into two (4") ramekins.

2. In a small microwave-safe pan, combine cream cheese, buffalo sauce, and Cheddar. Microwave for 20 seconds and then stir. Put a spoonful into each ramekin on top of the eggs.

3. Place ramekins into the fryer basket.

4. Set the temperature to 320°F and timer for 15 mins.

5. Serve warm.

Nutritional Value

- Calories: 354

- Protein: 20grams

- Fiber: 0.0grams

- Net Carbohydrates : 2.3grams

- Fat: 22.3grams

- Sodium: 886 mg

- Carbohydrates: 2.3grams

- sugar: 4grams

5. Veggie Frittata

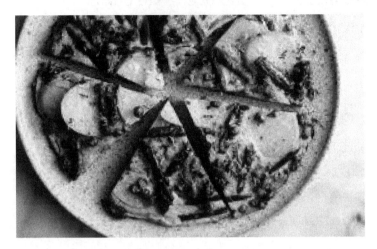

(Hands On Time: 15 minutes| Cook Time: 12 mins | Servings 1)

Things We Need

- Six large eggs
- 1/4 mug heavy whipping cream
- 1/2 mug chopped broccoli
- 1/4 mug chopped yellow onion
- 1/4mug chopped green bell pepper

Directions

1. In a large pan, whisk eggs and heavy whipping cream. Combine in broccoli, onion, and bell pepper.

2. Put into a 6" round oven-safe baking dish. Put the baking dish basket on the air fryer.

3. To adjust the temperature to 350°F and set the timer for 12 mins.

4. Eggs should be firm and cooked fully when the frittata is done.

5. Serve warm.

Nutritional Value

● Calories: 168

● Protein: 10.2grams

● Fiber: 0.6grams

● Net Carbohydrates : 2.5grams

● Fat: 18grams

● Sodium: 116 mg

● Carbohydrates: 3.1grams

● sugar: 5grams

6. Pumpkin Spice Muffins

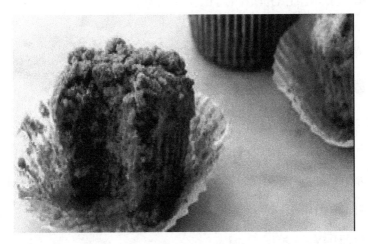

(Hands On Time: 10 minutes| Cook Time: 15 mins | Servings 6)

Things We Need

- One mug blanched finely ground almond flour

- 1/2 mug granular erythritol

- 1/2 tsp. baking powder

- 1/4 mug unsalted butter, softened

- 1/4 mug pure pumpkin purée

- 1/2 tsp. ground cinnamon

- 1/4 tsp. ground nutmeg

- 1 tsp. vanilla extract.

- Two large eggs

Directions

1. In a pan, combine almond flour, erythritol, baking powder, butter, pumpkin purée, cinnamon, nutmeg, and vanilla.

2. Gently mix in eggs.

3. Evenly put the batter into six silicone muffin mugs. Put muffin mugs into the air fryer basket, working in batches if necessary.

4. Adjust the temperature to 300°F and set the timer for 15 mins.

5. When thoroughly cooked, a toothpick inserted in the center will come out mostly clean. Serve warm.

Nutritional Value

- Calories: 205

- Protein: 6.3grams

- Fiber: 2.4grams

- Net Carbohydrates: 3.0grams

- sugar ALCOHOL: 12.0grams

- Fat: 18.0grams

- Sodium: 65 mg

- Carbohydrates: 17.4grams

- sugar: 3grams

Lunch

7. Quick Chicken Fajitas

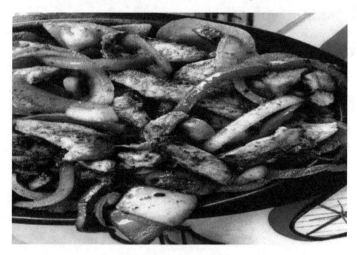

(Hands On Time: 10 minutes| Cook Time: 15 mins | Servings 2)

Things We Need

- 10 ounces boneless, skinless chicken breast, sliced into

- 1/4" strips

- 2 tbsp. coconut oil, melted

- one tablespoon chili powder

- 1/2 tsp. cumin
- 1/2 tsp. paprika
- 1/2 tsp. garlic powder
- 1/4 medium onion, peeled and sliced
- 1/2 medium green bell pepper, seeded and sliced
- 1/2 medium red bell pepper, seeded and sliced

Directions

1. Put chicken and coconut oil into a large pan and sprinkle with chili powder, cumin, paprika, and garlic powder. Toss chicken until well coated with seasoning. Put the chicken in the basket of the air fryer.
2. Set the temperature to 350°F and set the timer for 15 mins.
3. Add onion and peppers into the fryer basket when the timer has 7 mins remaining.
4. Toss the chicken two or three times during cooking. Vegetables should be tender and chicken fully cooked
5. To at least 165°F internal temperature when finished.
6. Serve warm.

Nutritional Value

- Calories: 326

- Protein: 33.5grams

- Fiber: 3.2grams

- Net Carbohydrates : 5.2gramsFat: 15.9grams

- Sodium: 180 mg

- Carbohydrates: 8.4grams

- sugar: 3.2grams

8. Chicken Patties

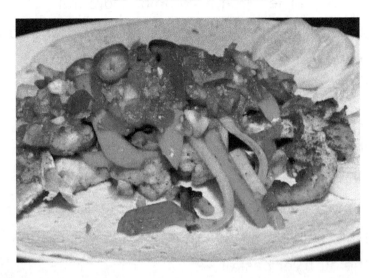

(Hands On Time: 15 minutes| Cook Time: 12 mins | Servings 4)

Things We Need

- 1 pound ground chicken thigh meat
- 1/2 mug shredded mozzarella cheese
- 1 tsp. dried parsley
- 1/2 tsp. garlic powder
- 1/4 tsp. onion powder one large egg
- 2 ounces pork rinds, finely ground

Directions

1. In a large pan, combine ground chicken, mozzarella, parsley, garlic powder, and onion powder. Form into four patties.
2. Put patties in the freezer for 15–20 mins until they begin to firm up.
3. Whisk egg in a medium pan. Put the ground pork rinds into a large pan.
4. Dip each chicken patty into the egg and then press into pork rinds to fully coat. Put patties into the air fryer basket.
5. To set, adjust the temperature to 360°F and set the timer for 12 mins.
6. Patties will be firm and cooked to an internal temperature of 165°F when done. Serve immediately.

Nutritional Value

- Calories: 304
- Protein: 32.7grams
- Fiber: 0.1grams
- Net Carbohydrates : 0.8gramsFat: 17.4grams
- Sodium: 406 mg

- Carbohydrates: 0.9gramssugar: 0.2grams

9. Greek Chicken Stir-Fry

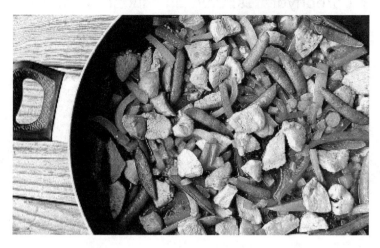

Hands on Time: 15 mins | Cook Time: 15 mins |Serving 2

Things We Need

- 1 (6-ounce) chicken breast, and cut into 1" cubes

- 1/2 medium zucchini, chopped

- 1/2 medium red bell pepper, seeded and chopped

- 1/4 medium red onion, peeled and sliced

- one tablespoon coconut oil

- 1 tsp. dried oregano

- 1/2 tsp. garlic powder

- 1/4 tsp. dried thyme

Directions

1. Put all ingredients into a large mixing pan and toss until the coconut oil coats the meat and vegetables. Put the contents of the pan.

2. To adjust the temperature to 375°F and set the timer for 15 mins.

3. To shake the fryer basket halfway through the cooking time to redistribute the food. Serve immediately.

Nutritional Value

- Calories: 186

- Protein: 20.4grams

- Fiber: 7grams

- Net Carbohydrates: 3.9grams

- Fat: 8.0grams

- Sodium: 43 mg

- Carbohydrates: 5.6grams

- sugar: 3.1grams

10. Chicken, Spinach, and Feta Bites

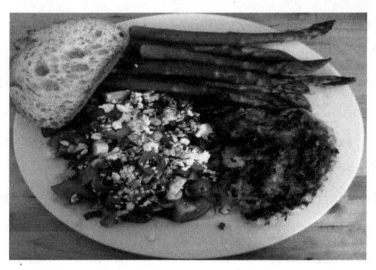

Hands on Time: 10 mins Cook Time: 12 mins | Serving 4

Things We Need

- 1 pound ground chicken thigh meat

- 1/3 mug frozen spinach, thawed and drained

- 1/3 mug crumbled feta

- 1/4 tsp. onion powder

- 1/2 tsp. garlic powder

- 1/2 ounce pork rinds, finely ground

How to start

1. Combine all ingredients in a large pan. Roll into 2" balls and put into the air fryer basket, working in batches if needed.
2. To set the temperature of the oven on 350°F and for 12 mins.
3. When done, the internal temperature will be 165°F.
4. Serve immediately.

PER SERVING

- Calories: 220
- Protein: 24.1grams
- Fiber: 0.4grams
- Net Carbohydrates: 1grams
- Fat: 12.2grams
- Sodium: 250 mg
- Carbohydrates: 5grams

- sugar: 0.6grams

11. Buffalo Chicken Cheese Sticks

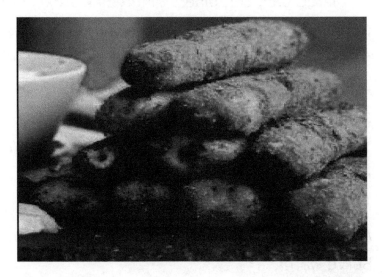

Hands on Time: 5 mins | Cook Time: 8 mins | Serving 2

Things We Need

- One mug shredded cooked chicken

- 1/4 mug buffalo sauce

- one mug shredded mozzarella cheese

- one large egg

- 1/4 mug crumbled feta

How to start

1. In a large pan, combine all ingredients except the feta. Cut a piece of parchment according to the air fryer basket's size and press the batter into a 1/2" -thick circle.
2. Sprinkle the batter with feta and put it into it.
3. To set the temperature on 400°F and timer for 8 mins.
4. After 5 mins, flip over the cheese batter.
5. Allow cooling 5 mins before cutting into sticks.
6. Serve warm.

PER SERVING

- Calories: 369
- Protein: 35.7gramsFiber: 0.0 g
- Net Carbohydrates : 2.2gramsFat: 25 g
- Sodium: 1,530 mg

- Carbohydrates: 2.2grams

- sugar: 4grams

12. Italian Chicken Thighs

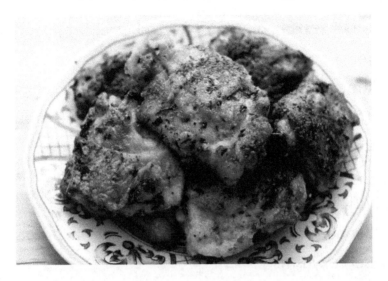

Hands on Time: 5 mins | Cook Time: 20 mins | Serving 2

Things We Need

- Four bone-in, skin-on chicken thighs 2 tbsp. unsalted butter, melted.
- 1 tsp. dried parsley
- 1 tsp. dried basil
- 1/2 tsp. garlic powder
- 1/4 tsp. onion powder
- 1/4 tsp. dried oregano

Directions

1. Brush chicken thighs with butter and sprinkle remaining ingredients over thighs. Put thighs into the air fryer basket.

2. To adjust the temperature to 380°F and timer for 20 mins.

3. Halfway through the cooking time, flip the thighs.

4. When fully cooked, the internal temperature will be at least 165°F, and the skin will be crispy. Serve warm.

PER SERVING

- Calories: 596
- Protein: 68.3grams
- Fiber: 0.4grams
- Net Carbohydrates: 0.8grams
- Fat: 30.9grams
- Sodium: 292 mg
- Carbohydrates: 2grams
- sugar: 0.1grams

13. Reverse Seared Rib eye

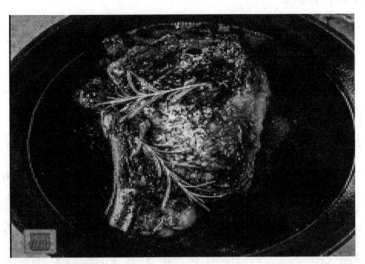

Hands on Time: 5 mins | Cook Time: 45 mins | Serving 2

Things We Need

- 1 (8-ounce) rib eye steak
- 1/2 tsp. pink Himalayan salt
- 1/4 tsp. ground peppercorn one tablespoon coconut oil
- One tablespoon salted butter softened
- 1/4 tsp. garlic powder
- 1/2 tsp. dried parsley
- 1/4 tsp. dried oregano.

How to start

1. Rub steak with salt and ground peppercorn. Put into the air fryer basket.
2. Adjust the temperature to 250°F and set the timer for 45 mins.
3. After the timer beeps, begin checking doneness and add a few mins until internal temperature is your personal preference.
4. In medium heat, add coconut oil. When the oil is hot, quickly sear outside and sides of the steak until crisp and browned. Transfer from heat and allow steak to rest.
5. In a small pan, whip butter with garlic powder, parsley, and oregano.
6. Slice steak and serve with herb butter on top.

PER SERVING

- Calories: 377
- Protein: 22.6grams
- Fiber: 0.2grams
- Net Carbohydrates : 0.4grams
- Fat: 30.7grams

- Sodium: 490 mg

- Carbohydrates: 0.6grams

- sugar: 0.0grams

SHORT ON TIME?

You can also quick-cook your rib eye! Put it into the air fryer at 400°F for 10–15 mins, depending on your preference for doneness. Don't forget to flip halfway through!

14. Pub-Style Burger

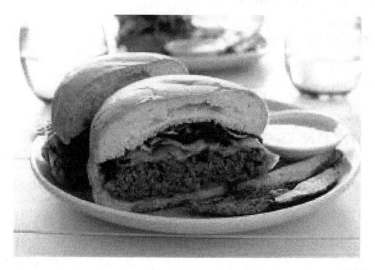

Hands on Time: 10 mins | Cook Time: 10 mins | Serving 4

Things We Need

- 1 pound ground sirloin
- Half tsp. salt, 1/4 tsp. ground black pepper
- 2 tbsp. salted butter, melted
- 1/2 mug full-Fat mayonnaise
- 2 tsp. sriracha.
- 1/4 tsp. garlic powder eight large leaves butter lettuce

- 4 Bacon-Wrapped Onion Rings (Chapter 3) 8 slices pickle

How to start

1. In a medium pan, combine ground sirloin, salt, and pepper. Form four patties. Brush each with butter and then put into the air fryer basket.

2. Adjust the temperature to 380°F and set the timer for 10 mins.

3. To flip the patties halfway through the cooking time for a medium burger. Add 3–5 mins for well-done.

4. In a small pan, combine mayonnaise, sriracha, and garlic powder. Set aside.

5. Put each cooked burger on a lettuce leaf and top with an onion ring, two pickles, and a dollop of your prepared burger sauce. Wrap another lettuce leaf around tightly to hold. Serve warm.

PER SERVING

- Calories: 442
- Protein: 22.3grams
- Fiber: 0.8grams
- Net Carbohydrates : 3.3grams
- Fat: 34.9grams

- Sodium: 928 mg
- Carbohydrates: 4.1grams

- sugar: 2.3grams

15. Pigs in a Blanket

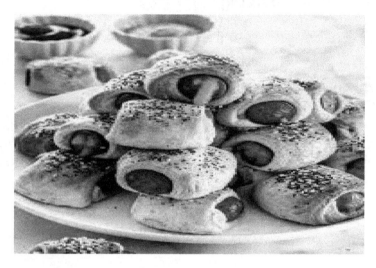

Hands on Time: 10 mins | Cook Time: 7 mins | Serving 2

Things We Need

- 1/2 mug shredded mozzarella cheese

- 2 tbsp. blanched finely ground almond flour

- 1-ounce full-Fat cream cheese
- 2 (2-ounce) beef smoked sausages
- 1/2 tsp. sesame seeds

How to Start

1. Put mozzarella, almond flour, and cream cheese in a large microwave-safe pan. Microwave it for 45 seconds and mix until smooth. Roll dough into a ball and cut in half.
2. Press each half out into a 4" × 5" rectangle. Roll one sausage up in each dough half and press seams closed. Sprinkle the top with sesame seeds.
3. Put each wrapped sausage into the air fryer basket.
4. To set the temperature at 400°F and set the timer for 7 mins.
5. The outside will be golden when thoroughly cooked.
6. Serve immediately.

PER SERVING

- Calories: 405
- Protein: 17.5grams
- Fiber: 0.8grams
- Net Carbohydrates : 2.1grams
- Fat: 32.2grams

- Sodium: 693 mg

- Carbohydrates: 2.9grams

- sugar: 0grams

16. Crispy Beef and Broccoli Stir-Fry

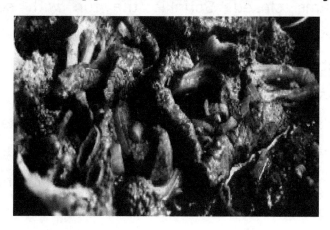

Hands on Time: 1 hour | Cook Time: 20 mins | Serving 2

Things We Need

- 1/2 pound sirloin steak, thinly sliced

- 2 tbsp. soy sauce (or liquid aminos)

- 1/4 tsp. grated ginger

- 1/4 tsp. finely minced garlic one tablespoon coconut oil
- Two mugs broccoli florets
- 1/4 tsp. crushed red pepper
- 1/8 tsp. xanthan gum
- 1/2 tsp. sesame seeds

How to start

1. To marinate beef, put it into a large pan or storage bag and add soy sauce, ginger, garlic, and coconut oil. Allow marinating for 1 hour in the refrigerator.
2. Transferable from marinade, reserving marinade and put beef into the basket of the air fryer.
3. Set the temperature to 320°F and set the timer for 20 mins.
4. After 10 mins, add broccoli and sprinkle red pepper into the fryer basket and shake.
5. Put the marinade into a skillet over medium heat and bring to a boil, then reduce to simmer. Mixing xanthan gum and allow it to thicken.
6. When the air fryer timer beeps, quickly empty the fryer basket into skillet and toss. Sprinkle with sesame seeds.
7. Serve immediately.

PER SERVING

- Calories: 342
- Protein: 27.0grams
- Fiber: 2.7grams

- Net Carbohydrates : 6.9gramsFat: 18.9grams

- Sodium: 418 mg

- Carbohydrates: 9.6grams

- sugar: 6grams

17. Empanadas

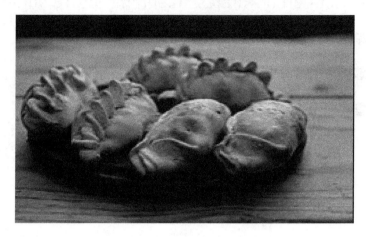

Hands on Time: 15 mins | Cook Time: 10 mins | 1 per serving

Things We Need

- 1 pound 80/20 ground beef
- 1/4 mug water 1/4 mug diced onion 2 tsp. powder of chili
- 1/2 tsp. powder of garlic,1/4 tsp. cumin, 11/2 mugs shredded mozzarella cheese 1/2 mug blanched finely ground almond flour 2 ounces full-Fat cream cheese
- One large egg

How to start

1. In medium heat, brown the ground beef for about 7–10 mins. Drain the Fat. Return skillet to stove.
2. Add water and onion to the skillet. Mix and sprinkle with chili powder, garlic powder, and cumin. Reduce heat and simmer an additional 3–5 mins. Transfer from heat and set aside.
3. In a large microwave-safe pan, add mozzarella, almond flour, and cream cheese—microwave for 1 minute. Mix until smooth. Form the batter into a ball.
4. Put dough between two sheets of parchment and roll out to 1/4" thickness. Cut the dough into four.
5. Squares. Put 1/4 of ground beef onto the bottom half of each square. Fold the dough over and roll the edges up or press with a wet fork to close.
6. Crack the egg into a small pan and whisk—brush egg over empanadas.
7. Cut a piece of parchment according to the air fryer basket's size and put the empanadas on the parchment. Put it on the fryer basket.
8. To adjust the temperature to 400°F and set the timer for 10 mins.

9. Flip the empanadas halfway through the cooking time.
10. Serve warm.

PER SERVING

- Calories: 463

- Protein: 33.3grams

- Fiber: 2.2grams

- Net Carbohydrates : 4.3grams

- Fat: 30.8grams

- Sodium: 426 mg

- Carbohydrates: 6.5grams

- sugar: 9grams

18. Peppercorn-Crusted Beef Tenderloin

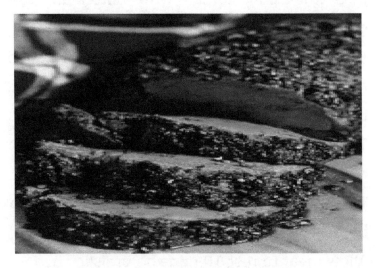

Hands on Time: 10 mins | Cook Time: 25 mins | Serving 6

Things We Need

- 2 tbsp. salted butter, melted

- 2 tsp. minced roasted garlic

- 3 tbsp. ground

- 4-peppercorn blend 1 (2-pound) beef tenderloin, trimmed of visible Fat

How to start

1. In a small pan, combine the butter and roasted garlic. Brush it over the beef tenderloin.
2. Put the ground peppercorns onto a plate and roll the tenderloin through them, creating a crust. Put tenderloin into the fryer-basket.
3. To adjust the temperature to 400°F and set the timer for 25 mins.
4. Turn the tenderloin halfway through the cooking time.
5. Allow meat to rest 10 mins before slicing.

PER SERVING

- Calories: 289
- Protein: 34.7grams
- Fiber: 0.9grams
- Net Carbohydrates : 6grams
- Fat: 13.8grams
- Sodium: 96 mg
- Carbohydrates: 2.5grams

- sugar: 0.0grams

19. Breaded Pork Chops

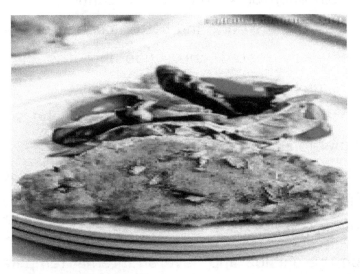

Hands on Time: 10 mins | Cook Time: 15 mins | Serving 4

Things We Need

- 11/2 ounces pork rinds, finely ground

- 1 tsp. chili powder

- 1/2 tsp. garlic powder

- one tablespoon coconut oil, melted

- 4 (4-ounce) pork chops

How to start

1. In a large pan, combine ground pork rinds, chili powder, and garlic powder.

2. Brush each pork chop with coconut oil and then press into the pork rind batter, coating both sides. Put each coated pork chop into the air fryer basket.
3. To adjust the temperature to 400°F and set the timer for 15 mins.
4. Flip each pork chop halfway through the cooking time.
5. When fully cooked, the pork chops will be golden on the outside and have an internal temperature of at least 145°F.

PER SERVING

- Calories: 292
- Protein: 29.5grams
- Fiber: 0.3grams
- Net Carbohydrates : 0.3grams
- Fat: 18.5grams
- Sodium: 268 mg
- Carbohydrates: 0.6grams

- sugar: 0.1grams

20. Easy Lasagna Casserole

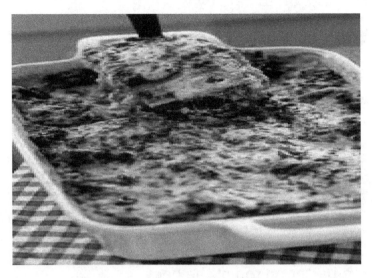

Hands on Time: 15 mins | Cook Time: 15 mins | Serving 4

Things We Need

- 3/4 mug low-carb no-sugar-added pasta sauce

- 1 pound 80/20 ground beef, cooked and drained

- 1/2 mug full-Fat ricotta cheese

- 1/4 mug grated Parmesan cheese

- 1/2 tsp. garlic powder

- 1 tsp. dried parsley
- 1/2 tsp. dried oregano one mug shredded mozzarella cheese

How to start

1. In a 4-mug round baking dish, put 1/4 mug of pasta sauce on the bottom of the dish. 1/4 of the ground beef put on top of the sauce.
2. In a small pan, combine ricotta, Parmesan, garlic powder, parsley, and oregano. Put dollops of half the batter on top of the beef.
3. Sprinkle with 1/3 of the mozzarella. Repeat layers
4. Until all beef, ricotta batter, sauce, and mozzarella are used, ending with the mozzarella.
5. To cover the dish with foil and put it fryer basket.
6. To adjust the temperature to 370°F and set the timer for 15 mins.
7. In the last 2 mins of cooking, transfer the foil to brown the cheese.
8. Serve immediately.

PER SERVING

- Calories: 371
- Protein: 34grams

- Fiber: 6grams

- Net Carbohydrates : 4.2grams

- Fat: 24grams

- Sodium: 633 mg

- Carbohydrates: 5.8grams

- sugar: 9grams

21. Fajita Flank Steak Rolls

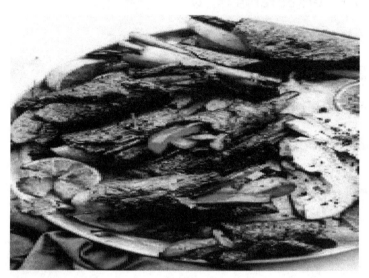

Hands on Time: 20 mins | Cook Time: 15 mins | Serving 6

Things We Need

- 2 tbsp. unsalted butter
- 1/4 mug diced yellow onion one medium red bell pepper, seeded and sliced into strips one medium green bell pepper, seeded and cut into strips 2 tsp. chili powder
- 1 tsp. cumin
- 1/2 tsp. garlic powder 2 pounds flank steak
- 4 (1-ounce) slices of pepper jack cheese

How to start

1. In medium heat, melt butter and begin sautéing onion, red bell pepper, and green bell pepper. Sprinkle with chili powder, cumin, and garlic powder. Sauté until peppers are tender, about 5–7 mins.

2. Lay flank steak flat on a work surface. Spread onion and pepper batter over the entire steak rectangle. Lay slices of cheese on top of onions and peppers, barely overlapping.

3. With the shortest end toward you, begin rolling the steak, tucking the cheese down into the roll as necessary. Secure the roll with twelve toothpicks, six on each side of the steak roll. Put steak roll into the air fryer basket.

4. To adjust the temperature to 400°F and set the timer for 15 mins.

5. Rotate the roll halfway through the cooking time. Add 1–4 mins depending on your preferred internal temperature (135°F for medium).

6. When the timer beeps, allow the roll to rest 15 mins, then slice into six even pieces.

7. Serve warm.

PER SERVING

- Calories: 439

- Protein: 38.0grams

- Fiber: 2grams

- Net Carbohydrates : 2.5grams

- Fat: 26.6grams

- Sodium: 226 mg

- Carbohydrates: 3.7grams

- sugar: 8gram

22. Cilantro Lime Baked Salmon

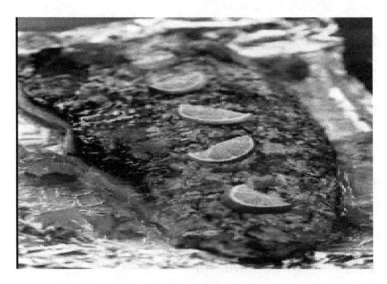

Whether you haven't cooked fish before or have been cooking it for years, this is a great staple recipe. The cilantro adds a freshness that is complemented well by the tartness of the lime. Try this dish with riced cauliflower or steamed veggies, and everyone will be asking for seconds.

Hands on Time: 10 mins | Cook Time: 12 mins | Serving 2

Things We Need

- 2 (3-ounce) salmon fillets, skin removed

- one tablespoon salted butter, melted

- 1 tsp. chili powder
- 1/2 tsp. minced garlic
- 1/4 mug sliced pickled jalapeños
- 1/2 medium lime, juiced
- 2 tbsp. chopped cilantro

How to start

1. After Brushing each salmon with butter and sprinkle with chili powder and garlic, put it into the 6'' round baking pan.
2. Put jalapeño slices on top and around salmon. Half of the lime juice put over the salmon. And cover it with foil. Then place into the fryer basket.
3. To adjust the temperature to 370°F and set the timer for 12 mins.
4. After fully cooked, salmon should flake easily with a fork's help and come back at an internal temperature of 145°F.
5. And then to serve, spritz with remaining lime juice and garnish with cilantro.

PER SERVING

- Calories: 167

- Protein: 15.8gram

- Fiber: 0.7gram

- Net Carbohydrates : 0.9grams

- Fat: 9.9gram

- Sodium: 248 mg

- Carbohydrates: 6grams

- sugar: 0.2gram

23. Sesame-Crusted Tuna Steak

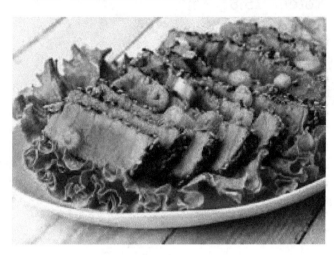

Hands on Time: 5 mins | Cook Time: 8 mins | Serving 2

Things We Need

- 2 (6-ounce) tuna steaks
- One tablespoon coconut oil melted
- 1/2 tsp. garlic powder
- 2 tsp. white sesame seeds
- 2 tsp. black sesame seeds

How to start

1. Brush each tuna steak with coconut oil and sprinkle with garlic powder.

2. In a large pan, combine sesame seeds and then press each tuna steak into them, covering the steak as completely as possible. Put tuna steaks in it.
3. To adjust the temperature to 400°F and set the timer for 8 mins.
4. Flip the steaks halfway through the cooking time. Steaks will be well-done at 145°F internal temperature.
5. Serve warm.

PER SERVING

- Calories: 280
- Protein: 42.7gram
- Fiber: 0.8gram
- Net Carbohydrates : 2grams
- Fat: 10.0gram
- Sodium: 77 mg
- Carbohydrates: 2.0grams

- sugar: 0.0gram

24. Spicy Salmon Jerky

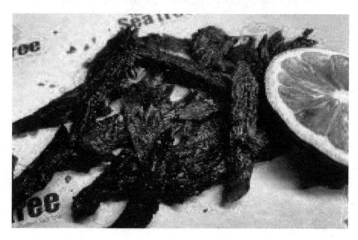

Hands on Time: 5 mins |Cook Time: 4 hours | Serving 4

Things We Need

- 1 pound salmon, skin and bones removed

- 1/4 mug soy sauce (or liquid aminos)

- 1/2 tsp. liquid smoke

- 1/4 tsp. ground black pepper Juice of 1/2 medium lime

- 1/2 tsp. ground ginger

- 1/4 tsp. red pepper flakes
- Slice salmon into 1/4"-thick slices, 4" long.

How to start

1. Put strips into a large storage bag or a covered pan and add the remaining ingredients. Allow marinating for 2 hours in the refrigerator.

2. Put each strip into the air fryer basket in a single layer.

3. Adjust the temperature to 140°F and set the timer for 4 hours.

4. First, Cool, then store in a sealed container until ready to eat.

PER SERVING

- Calories: 108
- Protein: 15.1gram
- Fiber: 0.2gram
- Net Carbohydrates : 0.8grams
- Fat: 4.1gram
- Sodium: 469 mg
- Carbohydrates: 0grams

- sugar: 0.1gram

25. Shrimp Kebabs

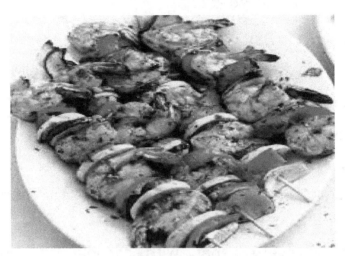

Hands on Time: 10 mins | Cook Time: 7 mins | Serving 2

Things We Need

- 18 medium shelled and deveined shrimp one medium zucchini, cut into 1" cubes

- 1/2 medium red bell pepper, cut into 1"-thick squares

- 1/4 medium red onion, cut into 1"-thick squares

- 11/2 tbsp. coconut oil, melted

- 2 tsp. chili powder
- 1/2 tsp. paprika
- 1/4 tsp. ground black pepper

How to start

1. For 30 mins soak four 6" bamboo skewers in water. Put a shrimp on the skewer, then a zucchini, a pepper, and an onion. Repeat until all ingredients are utilized.
2. Brush every kebab with coconut oil and put kebabs into the air fryer basket.
3. To adjust the temperature to 400°F and set the timer for 7 mins or until shrimp is fully cooked and veggies are tender.
4. Flip kebabs do halfway through the cooking time.
5. Serve warm.

PER SERVING

- Calories: 166
- Protein: 9.5gram
- Fiber: 3.1gram
- Net Carbohydrates : 5.4grams
- Fat: 10.7gram

- Sodium: 391 mg

- Carbohydrates: 8.5grams

- sugar: 4.5gram

26. Simple Buttery Cod

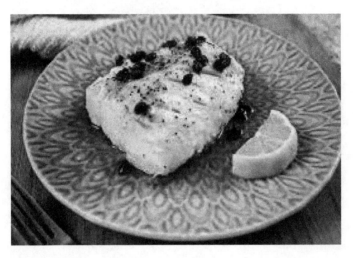

This is a delicious and simple recipe that's a perfect weeknight staple. To make sure this dish is full of buttery flavor, buy quality butter. Irish butter, such as Kerry gold, is deeper in color and has a much richer flavor than a store–brand butter.

Hands on Time: 5 mins | Cook Time: 8 mins |Serving 2

Things We Need

- 2 (4-ounce) cod fillets

- 2 tbsp. salted butter, melted

- 1 tsp. Old Bay seasoning

- 1/2 medium lemon, sliced

How to start

1. Put cod fillets into a 6" round baking dish. Brush each fillet with butter and sprinkle with Old Bay seasoning. Lay two lemon slices on each fillet. To cover foil, put it into the air fryer basket.

2. To adjust the temperature to 350°F and set the timer for 8 mins.

3. Flip halfway through the cooking time. When cooked, the internal temperature should be at least 145°F.

4. Serve warm.

PER SERVING

- Calories: 179

- Protein: 17.4grams

- Fiber: 0.0gram

- Net Carbohydrates : 0.0grams

- Fat: 11gram

- Sodium: 714 mg

- Carbohydrates: 0.0grams

- sugar: 0.0gram

27. Spicy Parmesan Artichokes

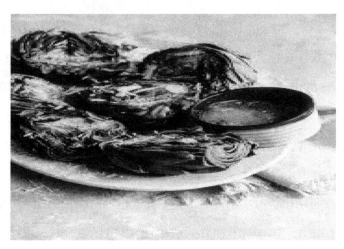

Hands on Time: 10 mins | Cook Time: 10 mins | Serving 4

Things We Need

- Two medium artichokes, trimmed and quartered, center removed

- 2 tbsp. coconut oil.

- One large egg, beaten.

- 1/2 mug grated vegetarian Parmesan cheese

- 1/4 mug blanched finely ground almond flour

- 1/2tsp crushed red pepper flakes

How to start

1. In a large pan, toss artichokes in coconut oil and then dip each piece into the egg.
2. Combine the Parmesan and almond flour in a large pan. Add artichoke pieces and toss to cover as completely as possible, sprinkle with pepper flakes. Put into the air fryer basket.
3. To adjust the temperature to 400°F and set the timer for 10 mins.
4. Toss the basket two times during cooking.
5. Serve warm.

PER SERVING

- Calories: 189
- Protein: 7.9gram
- Fiber: 4.2gram
- Net Carbohydrates : 5.8grams
- Fat: 13.5gram
- Sodium: 294 mg
- Carbohydrates: 10.0grams

- sugar: 0.9gram

28. Zucchini Cauliflower Fritters

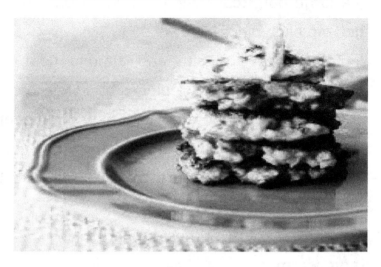

Hands on Time: 15 mins | Cook Time: 12 mins | Serving 2

Things We Need

- 1 (12-ounce) cauliflower steamer bag one medium zucchini, shredded
- 1/4 mug almond flour one large egg
- 1/2 tsp. garlic powder
- 1/4 mug grated vegetarian Parmesan cheese

How to start

1. Cook cauliflower according to package instructions and drain excess moisture in a cheesecloth or paper towel. Put into a large pan.

2. Put zucchini into the paper towel and pat down to transfer excess moisture. Add to pan with the cauliflower. Add remaining ingredients.

3. Divide the batter evenly and form four patties. Press into 1/4"-thick patties. Put each into the air fryer basket.

4. Adjust the temperature to 320°F and set the timer for 12 mins.

5. Fritters will be firm when fully cooked. Allow cooling 5 mins before moving. Serve warm.

PER SERVING

- Calories: 217
- Protein: 13.7gram
- Fiber: 6.5gram
- Net Carbohydrates : 8.5grams
- Fat: 12.0gram
- Sodium: 263 mg
- Carbohydrates: 16.1grams

- sugar: 6.8grams

29. Basic Spaghetti Squash

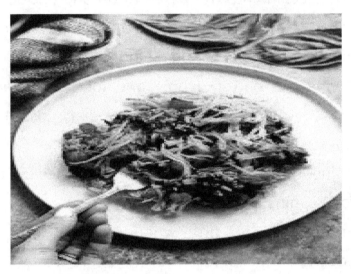

Hands on Time: 10 mins | Cook Time: 45 mins | Serving 2

Things We Need

- 1/2 large spaghetti squash

- one tablespoon coconut oil

- 2 tbsp. salted butter, melted

- 1/2 tsp. garlic powder 1

- tsp. dried parsley

How to start

1. Brush shell of spaghetti squash with coconut oil. Put the skin side down and brush the inside with

butter. Sprinkle with garlic powder and parsley.

2. Put squash with the skin side down in the fryer basket.

3. To adjust the temperature to 350°F and set the timer for 30 mins.

4. When the timer beeps, flip the squash so the skin side is up and cooks an additional 15 mins or until fork tender.

5. Serve warm.

PER SERVING

- Calories: 182

- Protein: 9gram

- Fiber: 3.9gram

- Net Carbohydrates : 14.3grams

- Fat: 17gram

- Sodium: 134 mg

- Carbohydrates: 18.2grams

- sugar: 7.0gram

30. Spaghetti Squash Alfredo

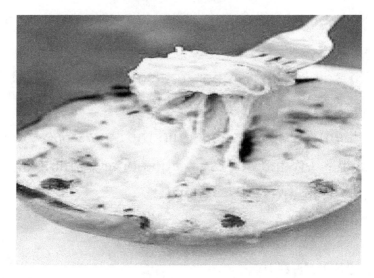

Hands on Time: 10 mins | Cook Time: 15 mins |Serving 2

Things We Need

- 1/2 large cooked spaghetti squash

- 2 tbsp. salted butter, melted

- 1/2 mug low-carb Alfredo sauce

- 1/4 mug grated vegetarian Parmesan cheese

- 1/2 tsp. garlic powder

- 1 tsp. dried parsley
- 1/4 tsp. ground peppercorn
- 1/2 mug shredded Italian blend cheese

How to start

1. Using a fork, transfer the strands of spaghetti squash from the shell. Put into a large pan with butter and Alfredo sauce. Sprinkle with Parmesan, garlic powder, parsley, and peppercorn.
2. Put into a 4-mug round baking dish and top with shredded cheese. Put the dish into the air fryer basket.
3. Adjust the temperature to 320°F and set the timer for 15 mins.
4. When finished, the cheese will be golden and bubbling.
5. Serve immediately.

PER SERVING

- Calories: 375
- Protein: 13.5gram
- Fiber: 4.0gram
- Net Carbohydrates : 20.1grams

- Fat: 24.2gram

- Sodium: 950 mg

- Carbohydrates: 24.1grams

31. Caprese Eggplant Stacks

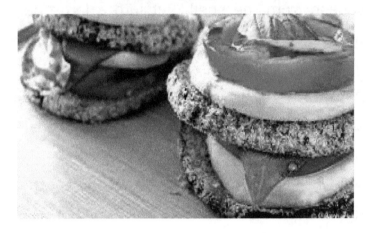

These stacks are a warm twist on the classic fresh Caprese salad.

Hands on Time: 5 mins |Cook Time: 12 mins | Serving 4

Things We Need

- One medium eggplant, cut into 1/4" slices

- two large tomatoes, cut into 1/4" slices

- 4 ounces fresh mozzarella, cut into 1/2-ounce slices

- 2 tbsp. olive oil.

- 1/4 mug fresh basil, sliced

How to start

1. In a 6" round baking dish, put four slices of eggplant on the bottom. Put the tomato on top of each eggplant round, then mozzarella, then eggplant. Repeat as necessary.
2. Drizzle with olive oil. Cover the dish with foil and put the dish into the air fryer basket.
3. To adjust the temperature to 350°F and set the timer for 12 mins.
4. When done, the eggplant will be tender. Garnish with fresh basil to serve.

PER SERVING

- Calories: 195
- Protein: 8.5gram
- Fiber: 5.2gram
- Net Carbohydrates : 7.5grams
- Fat: 12.7gram
- Sodium: 184 mg
- Carbohydrates: 12.7grams

- sugar: 7.5gram

32. Crust less Spinach Cheese Pie

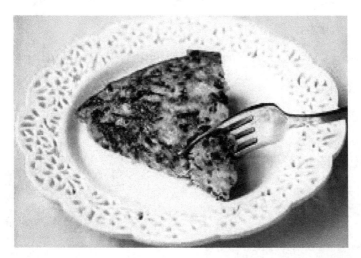

Hands on Time: 10 mins |Cook Time: 20 mins |Serving 4

Things We Need

- Six large eggs
- 1/4 mug heavy whipping cream
- one mug frozen chopped spinach, drained
- one mug shredded sharp Cheddar cheese
- 1/4 mug diced yellow onion

How to start

1. In a medium pan, whisk eggs and add cream. Add remaining ingredients to the pan.
2. Put into a 6" round baking dish.

3. To adjust the temperature to 320°F and set the timer for 20 mins.

4. Eggs will be firm and slightly browned when cooked.

5. Serve immediately.

PER SERVING

- Calories: 288

- Protein: 18.0gram

- Fiber: 3gram

- Net Carbohydrates : 2.6grams

- Fat: 20.0gram

- Sodium: 322 mg

- Carbohydrates: 3.9grams

- sugar: 5gram

33. Broccoli Crust Pizza

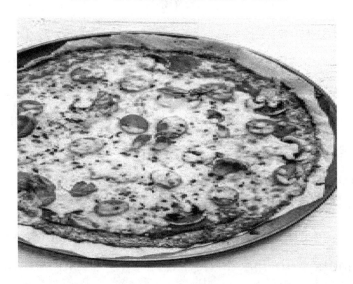

Hands on Time: 15 mins | Cook Time: 12 mins | Serving 4

Things We Need

- Three mugs riced broccoli, steamed, and drained well

- one large egg
- 1/2 mug grated vegetarian Parmesan cheese
- 3 tbsp. low-carb Alfredo sauce
- 1/2 mug shredded mozzarella cheese

How to start

1. In a large pan, combine broccoli, egg, and Parmesan.
2. Cut parchment to fit your fryer basket. Press out the pizza batter to fit on the parchment, working in two batches if necessary. Put into the air fryer basket.
3. To adjust the temperature to 370°F and set the timer for 5 mins.
4. When the timer beeps, the crust should be firm enough to flip. If not, add two additional mins— flip crust.
5. Top with Alfredo sauce and mozzarella. Return to the air fryer basket and cook for an additional 7 mins or until the cheese is golden and bubbling.
6. Serve warm.

PER SERVING

- Calories: 136
- Protein: 9.9grams
- Fiber: 2.3gram
- Net Carbohydrates : 3.4grams
- Fat: 7.6gram

- Sodium: 421 mg

- Carbohydrates: 5.7grams

- sugar: 1gram

34. Italian Baked Egg and Veggies

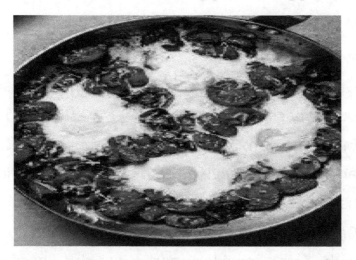

Hands on Time: 10 mins |Cook Time: 10 mins | Serving 2

Things We Need

- 2 tbsp. salted butter
- One small zucchini, sliced lengthwise and quartered

- 1/2 medium green bell pepper, seeded and diced
- One mug fresh spinach, chopped.
- One medium Roma tomato, diced
- Two large eggs
- 1/4 tsp. onion powder 1/4 tsp. garlic powder
- 1/2 tsp. dried basil 1/4tsp dried oregano

How to start

1. Grease two (4") ramekins with one tablespoon butter each.
2. In a large pan, toss zucchini, bell pepper, spinach, and tomatoes. Divide the batter into two and put half in each ramekin.
3. Crack an egg on top of each ramekin and sprinkle with onion powder, garlic powder, basil, and oregano. Put into the air fryer basket.
4. Adjust the temperature to 330°F and set the timer for 10 mins.
5. Serve immediately.

PER SERVING

- Calories: 150

- Protein: 8.3gram

- Fiber: 2.2gram

- Net Carbohydrates : 4.4grams

- Fat: 10.0gram

- Sodium: 135 mg

- Carbohydrates: 6.6gram

- sugar: 3.7gram

Dinner

35.   BBQ "Pulled" Mushrooms

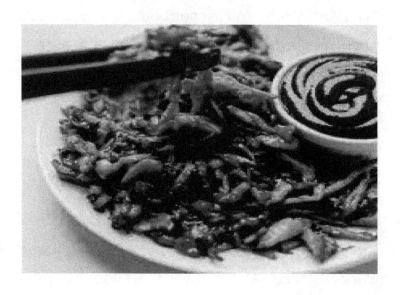

Hands on Time: 5 mins |Cook Time: 12 mins | Serving 2

Things We Need

- Four large Portobello mushrooms
- One tablespoon salted butter melted
- 1/4 tsp. ground black pepper
- 1 tsp. chili powder.
- 1 tsp. paprika
- 1/4 tsp. onion powder
- 1/2 mug low-carb, sugar-free barbecue sauce

How to start

1. Transfer stem and scoop out the underside of each mushroom. Brush the caps with butter and sprinkle with pepper, chili powder, paprika, and onion powder.
2. Put mushrooms into the air fryer basket.
3. To adjust the temperature to 400°F and set the timer for 8 mins.
4. When the timer beeps, transfer mushrooms from the basket and put them on a cutting board or work surface. Using two forks gently pull the

mushrooms apart, creating strands.

5. Put mushroom strands into a 4-mug round baking dish with barbecue sauce. Put the dish into the air fryer basket.

6. To adjust the temperature to 350°F and set the timer for 4 mins.

7. Mix halfway through the cooking time.

8. Serve warm.

PER SERVING

- Calories: 108

- Protein: 3.3gram

- Fiber: 2.7gram

- Net Carbohydrates : 8.2grams

- Fat: 5.9gram

- Sodium: 476 mg

- Carbohydrates: 10.9grams

- sugar: 3.6gram

36.   Mozzarella-Stuffed Meatballs

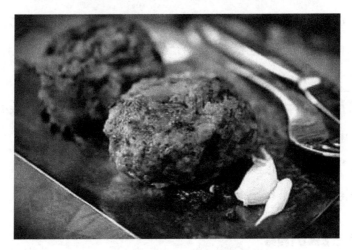

Hands on Time: 15 mins |Cook Time: 15 mins | Yields 16 meatballs (4 per serving)

Things We Need

- 1 pound 80/20 ground beef
- 1/4 mug blanched finely ground almond flour
- 1 tsp. dried parsley
- 1/2 tsp. garlic powder 1/4 tsp. onion powder one large egg
- 3 ounces low-moisture, whole-milk mozzarella, cubed
- 1/2 mug low-carb, no-sugar-added pasta sauce
- 1/4 mug grated Parmesan cheese

How to start

1. In a large pan, add ground beef, almond flour, parsley, garlic powder, onion powder, and egg. Fold ingredients together until fully combined.

2. Form the batter into 2" balls and use your thumb or a spoon to create an indent in the center of each meatball. Put a cube of cheese in the center and form the ball around it.

3. Put the meatballs into the air fryer, working in batches if necessary.

4. To adjust the temperature to 350°F and set the timer for 15 mins.

5. Meatballs will be slightly crispy on the outside and fully cooked when at least 180°F internally.

6. When they are finished cooking, toss the meatballs in the sauce and sprinkle with grated Parmesan for serving.

PER SERVING

- Calories: 447
- Protein: 29.6gram
- Fiber: 8gram
- Net Carbohydrates : 3.6gramsFat: 29.7gram

- Sodium: 509 mg

- Carbohydrates: 5.4gram

- sugar: 6gram

INTERCHANGEABLE CHEESE!

You can customize this dish by swapping the mozzarella for your favorite cheese! For a taco-inspired meatball, add a packet of taco seasoning to your batter and use pepper jack or Cheddar cheese cubes for stuffing!

37. Ranch Roasted Almonds

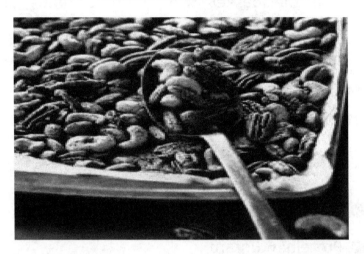

Hands on Time: 5 mins | Cook Time: 6 mins | Yields 2 mugs (1/4 mug per serving)

Things We Need

- Two mugs of raw almonds
- 2 tbsp. unsalted butter, melted
- 1/2 (1-ounce) ranch dressing \ packet

How to start

1. In a large pan, toss almonds in butter to evenly coat. Sprinkle ranch over almonds and toss. Put almonds into the air fryer basket.

2. To adjust the temperature to 320°F and set the timer for 6 mins.

3. Shake the basket two or three times during cooking.

4. Let cool for at least 20 mins. Almonds will be soft but become crunchier during cooling. Put this in an airtight container for up to 3 days.

PER SERVING

- Calories: 190
- Protein: 6.0gram
- Fiber: 3.0gram
- Net Carbohydrates : 4.0gramsFat: 16.7gram
- Sodium: 133 mg
- Carbohydrates: 7.0gramssugar: 0gram

38. Loaded Roasted Broccoli

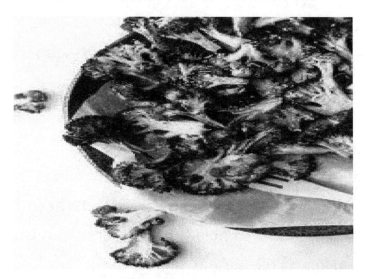

Hands on Time: 10 mins | Cook Time: 10 mins | Serving 2

Things We Need

- Three mugs fresh broccoli florets
- One tablespoon coconut oil
- 1/2 mug shredded sharp Cheddar cheese
- 1/4 mug full-Fat sour cream
- four slices sugar-free bacon, cooked and crumbled
- one scallion, sliced on the bias

How to start

1. Put broccoli into the air fryer basket and drizzle it with coconut oil.
2. To adjust the temperature to 350°F and set the timer for 10 mins.
3. Toss the basket two or three times during cooking to avoid burned spans.
4. When broccoli begins to crisp at ends, transfer from the fryer. Top with shredded cheese, sour cream, and crumbled bacon, and garnish with scallion slices.

PER SERVING

- Calories: 361
- Protein: 18.4gram
- Fiber: 3.6gram
- Net Carbohydrates : 6.9grams
- Fat: 25.7gram
- Sodium: 564 mg
- Carbohydrates: 10.5grams

- sugar: 3.3gram

39. Garlic Herb Butter Roasted Radishes

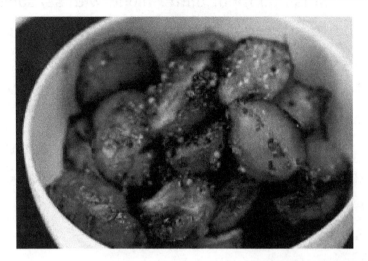

Hands on Time: 10 mins | Cook Time: 10 mins | Serving 4

Things We Need

- 1 pound radishes
- 2 tbsp. unsalted butter, melted
- 1/2 tsp. garlic powder
- 1/2 tsp. dried parsley
- 1/4tsp dried oregano
- 1/4 tsp. ground black pepper

How to start

1. Transfer roots from radishes and cut them into quarters.

2. In a small pan, put butter along with seasonings. And toss the radishes in the herb butter and put them into the air fryer basket.

3. To adjust the temperature to 350°F and set the timer for 10 mins.

4. In half of the cooking time, toss the radishes in the air fryer basket. Continue cooking until the edges begin to turn brown.

5. Serve warm.

PER SERVING

- Calories: 63
- Protein: 0.7grams
- Fiber: 3grams
- Net Carbohydrates : 6grams
- Fat: 5.4grams
- Sodium: 28 mg

- Carbohydrates: 2.9grams

- sugar: 4grams

40. Sausage-Stuffed Mushroom Caps

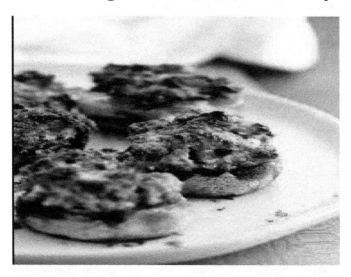

Hands on Time: 10 mins | Cook Time: 8 mins | Serving 2

Things We Need

- Six large Portobello mushroom caps

- 1/2 pound Italian sausage

- 1/4 mug chopped onion

- 2 tbsp. blanched finely ground almond flour

- 1/4 mug grated Parmesan cheese

● 1 tsp. minced fresh garlic.

How to start

1. Use a spoon to hollow out each mushroom cap, reserving scrapings.

2. In medium heat, brown the sausage about 10 mins or until fully cooked, and no pink remains. Drain and then add reserved mushroom scrapings, onion, almond flour, Parmesan, and garlic. Gently fold ingredients together and continue cooking for an additional minute, then transfer from heat.

3. Evenly spoon the batter into mushroom caps and put the lids into a 6" round pan.

4. To adjust the temperature to 375°F and set the timer for 8 mins.

5. When finished cooking, the tops will be browned and bubbling.

6. Serve warm.

PER SERVING

- Calories: 404
- Protein: 24.3grams
- Fiber: 4.5grams
- Net Carbohydrates : 13.7grams

- Fat: 25.8grams

- Sodium: 1,106 mg

- Carbohydrates: 18.2grams

- sugar: 8.1grams

41. Cheesy Cauliflower Tots

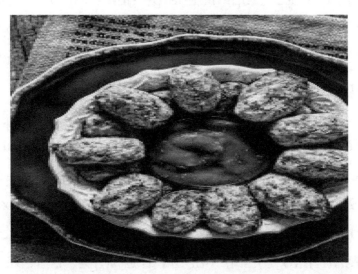

Hands on Time: 15 mins | Cook Time: 12 mins | Yields 16 tots (4 per serving)

Things We Need

- One large head cauliflower
- One mug shredded mozzarella cheese
- 1/2 mug Parmesan cheese
- One large egg
- 1/4 tsp. garlic powder
- 1/4 tsp. dried parsley
- 1/8 tsp. onion powder

How to start

1. On the stovetop, fill a large pan with two mugs of water and put a steamer in the pan. Bring water to a boil. To cut the cauliflower into florets and put it on a steamer basket—cover pan with lid.

2. Allow cauliflower to steam 7 mins until fork tender. Transfer from steamer basket and put into cheesecloth or clean kitchen towel and let cool. Squeeze over the sink to transfer as much excess moisture as possible. The batter will be too soft to form into tots if not all the water is removed. Mash with a fork to a smooth consistency.

3. Put the cauliflower into a large mixing pan and add mozzarella, Parmesan, egg, garlic powder, parsley, and onion powder. Mix until thoroughly combine d. The batter should be wet but easy to mold.

4. Take 2 tbsp. of the batter and roll into tot shape. Repeat with the remaining batter.

5. To set the temperature to 320°F and set the timer for 12 mins.

6. Turn tots halfway through the cooking time. Cauliflower tots should be golden when fully cooked.

7. Serve warm.

Per servings

- Calories: 181

- Protein: 13.5grams

- Fiber: 3.0grams

- Net Carbohydrates : 6.6gramsFat: 9.5grams

- Sodium: 417 mg

- Carbohydrates: 9.6gramssugar: 3.2grams

KID-FRIENDLY!

These are great to make for kids because they look just like a classic tater tot, but they're much better for you. The cheese also helps to mask the cauliflower taste, making this the ultimate way to sneak veggies in!

42.   Crispy Brussels sprouts

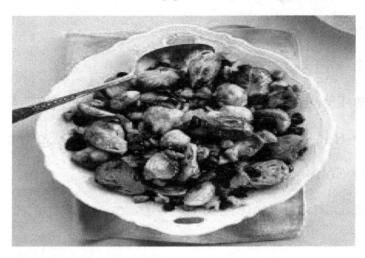

Hands on Time: 5 mins | Cook Time: 10 mins | Serving 4

Things We Need

- 1 pound Brussels sprouts

- one tablespoon coconut oil

- one tablespoon unsalted butter, melted

How to start

1. Transfer all loose leaves from Brussels sprouts and cut each in half.

2. Drizzle sprouts with coconut oil and put into the air fryer basket.

3. To adjust the temperature to 400°F and set the timer for 10 mins. You may want to gently mix throughout the cooking time until its color changes to brown.
4. After thoroughly cooked, they should be tender with darker caramelized spans. Transfer from the fryer basket and drizzle with melted butter.
5. Serve immediately.

PER SERVING

- Calories: 90
- Protein: 2.9grams
- Fiber: 3.2grams
- Net Carbohydrates : 4.3grams
- Fat: 6.1grams
- Sodium: 21 mg

- Carbohydrates: 7.5grams

- sugar: 9gram

43. Zucchini Parmesan Chips

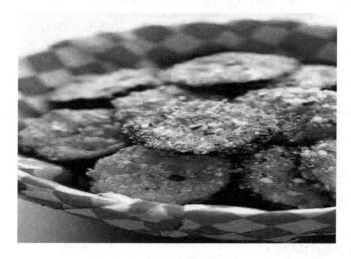

Hands on Time: 10 mins | Cook Time: 10 mins | Serving 4

Things We Need

- Two medium zucchini
- 1-ounce pork rinds
- 1/2 mug grated Parmesan cheese one large egg
- Slice zucchini in 1/4"-thick slices.

How to start

1. Put between the paper towels layers or a clean kitchen towel for 30 mins to transfer excess moisture.

2. Put pork rinds into the food processor and pulse until finely ground. Put into a medium pan and combine with Parmesan.

3. Beat egg in a small pan.

4. Dip zucchini slices in egg and then in pork rind batter, coating as completely as possible. Carefully put each piece into the air fryer basket in a single layer, working in batches as necessary.

5. Adjust temperature to 320°F and set the timer for 10 mins.

6. Flip chips do halfway through the cooking time.

7. Serve warm.

PER SERVING

- Calories: 121
- Protein: 9.9grams
- Fiber: 0.6grams
- Net Carbohydrates : 3.2grams
- Fat: 6.7grams
- Sodium: 364 mg

- Carbohydrates: 3.8grams

● sugar: 6grams

44. Roasted Garlic

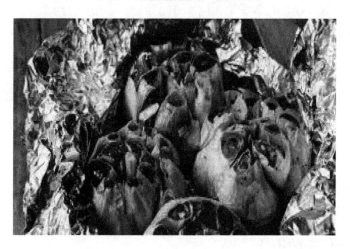

Hands on Time: 5 mins |Cook Time: 20 mins |Yields 12 cloves (1 per serving)

Things We Need

- One medium head garlic

- 2 tsp. avocado oil

How to start

1. Transfer any hanging excess peel from the garlic but leave the cloves covered. Cut off 1/4 of the head of garlic, exposing the tips of the cloves.

2. Drizzle with avocado oil. Put the garlic head into a small sheet of aluminum foil, completely enclosing it. Put into it.

3. To adjust the temperature to 400°F and set the timer for 20 mins. If your garlic head is a bit smaller, check it after 15 mins.

4. When done, garlic should be golden brown and very soft.

5. For the serving, cloves should pop out and easily be spread or sliced. Stored it into an airtight container in the refrigerator for up to 5 days. You may also freeze individual cloves on a baking sheet, and then store them together in a freezer-safe storage bag once frozen.

PER SERVING

- Calories: 11
- Protein: 0.2grams
- Fiber: 0.1grams
- Net Carbohydrates : 0.9grams
- Fat: 0.7grams
- Sodium: 0 mg

- Carbohydrates: 0grams

- sugar: 0.0grams

45. Kale Chips

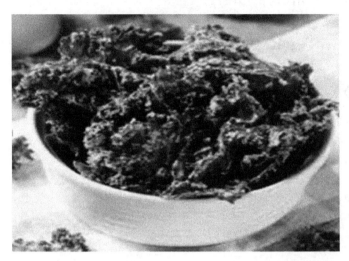

Hands on Time: 5 mins | Cook Time: 5 mins | Serving 4

Things We Need

- Four mugs stemmed kale.

- 2 tsp. avocado oil

- 1/2 tsp. salt

How to start

1. In a large pan, toss the kale in avocado oil and sprinkle with salt. Put into the air fryer basket.

2. To adjust the temperature to 400°F and set the timer for 5 mins.

3. Kale will be crispy when done.

4. Serve immediately.

PER SERVING

- Calories: 25

- Protein: 0.5grams

- Fiber: 0.4grams

- Net Carbohydrates : 0.7grams

- Fat: 2.2grams

- Sodium: 295 mg

- Carbohydrates: 1grams

- sugar: 0.3grams

46. Buffalo Cauliflower

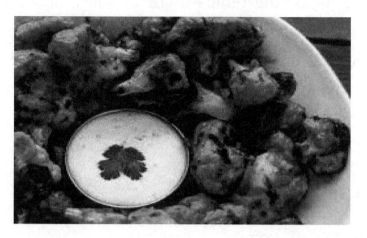

Hands on Time: 5 mins | Cook Time: 5 mins | Serving 4

Things We Need

- Four mugs cauliflower florets

- 2 tbsp. salted butter, melted

- 1/2 (1-ounce) dry ranch seasoning packet

- 1/4 mug buffalo sauce.

How to start

1. In a large pan, toss cauliflower with butter and dry ranch. Put into the air fryer basket.

2. To adjust the temperature to 400°F and set the timer for 5 mins.
3. Shake the basket two or three times during cooking. When tender, transfer cauliflower from the fryer basket and toss in buffalo sauce.
4. Serve warm.

PER SERVING

- Calories: 87
- Protein: 2.1grams
- Fiber: 2.1grams
- Net Carbohydrates : 5.2grams
- Fat: 5.6grams
- Sodium: 803 mg

- Carbohydrates: 7.3grams

- sugar: 2.1grams

47. Green Bean Casserole

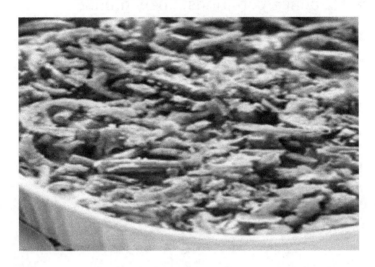

Hands on Time: 10 mins |Cook Time: 15 mins | Serving 4

Things We Need

- 4 tbsp. unsalted butter
- 1/4 mug diced yellow onion
- 1/2 mug chopped white mushrooms
- 1/2 mug heavy whipping cream 1-ounce full-Fat cream cheese
- 1/2 mug chicken broth
- 1/4 tsp. xanthan gum
- 1 pound fresh green beans, edges trimmed

- 1/2 ounce pork rinds, finely ground

How to start

1. In medium heat, melt the butter. Sauté the onion and mushrooms until they become soft and fragrant, about 3–5 mins.

2. Add the heavy whipping cream, cream cheese, and broth to the pan. Whisk until smooth. Bring to a boil and then reduce to a simmer. Spread the xanthan gum into the pan and transfer from heat.

3. Chop the green beans into 2" pieces and put them into a 4-mug round baking dish. Put the sauce batter over

4. Them and mix until coated. Top the dish with ground pork rinds. Put into the air fryer basket.

5. To adjust the temperature to 320°F and set the timer for 15 mins.

6. The top will be golden and green beans fork-tender when fully cooked. Serve warm.

PER SERVING

- Calories: 267
- Protein: 3.6grams
- Fiber: 3.2grams
- Net Carbohydrates : 6.5grams

- Fat: 23.4grams
- Sodium: 161 mg
- Carbohydrates: 9.7grams
- sugar: 5.1grams

48. Cilantro Lime Roasted Cauliflower

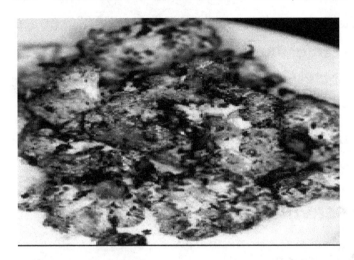

Hands on Time: 10 mins | Cook Time: 7 mins | Serving 4

Things We Need

● Two mugs chopped cauliflower florets

● 2 tbsp. coconut oil, melted

● 2 tsp. chili powder.

● 1/2 tsp. garlic powder one medium lime

● 2 tbsp. chopped cilantro

How to start

1. In a large pan, toss cauliflower with coconut oil. Sprinkle it with chili powder and garlic powder.

Put seasoned cauliflower on it.

2. To adjust the temperature to 350°F and set the timer for 7 mins.

3. Cauliflower will be tender and begin to turn golden at the edges. Put into serving pan.

4. Cut the lime into quarters and squeeze juice over cauliflower. Garnish with cilantro.

PER SERVING

- Calories: 73

- Protein: 1grams

- Fiber: 1grams

- Net Carbohydrates : 2.2grams

- Fat: 6.5grams

- Sodium: 16 mg

- Carbohydrates: 3.3grams

- sugar: 1grams

49. Dinner Rolls

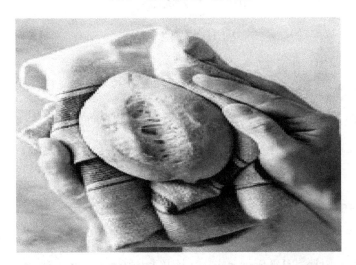

Do you miss bread on your keto diet? This low-carb substitute will satisfy any bread craving you may have and give you a great side dish to eat with your dinner. The dough can also be baked in a loaf pan or flattened out on a pizza pan to take care of you no matter which bread craving strikes!

Hands on Time: 10 mins | Cook Time: 12 mins | Serving 6

Things We Need

- One mug shredded mozzarella cheese 1-ounce full-Fat cream cheese
- One mug blanched finely ground almond flour

- 1/4 mug ground flaxseed
- 1/2 tsp. baking powder
- one large egg

How to start

1. Put mozzarella, cream cheese, and almond flour in a large microwave-safe pan—microwave for 1 minute. Combine until smooth.
2. Add flaxseed, baking powder, and egg until thoroughly combined and smooth. Microwave an additional 15 seconds if it becomes too firm.
3. Separate the dough into six pieces and roll it into balls. Put the balls into the air fryer basket.
4. Adjust the temperature to 320°F and set the timer for 12 mins.
5. Allow rolls to cool completely before serving.

PER SERVING

- Calories: 228
- Protein: 10.8grams
- Fiber: 3.9grams
- Net Carbohydrates : 2.9grams
- Fat: 18.1 g

- Sodium: 188 mg

- Carbohydrates: 6.8grams

- sugar: 2grams

50.   Coconut Flour Cheesy Garlic Biscuits

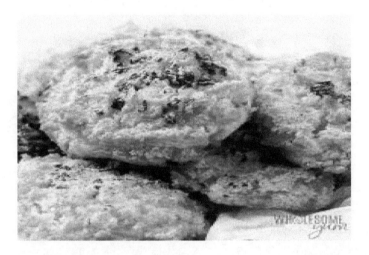

Hands on Time: 10 mins | Cook Time: 12 mins | Serving 4

Things We Need

- 1/3 mug coconut flour

- 1/2 tsp. baking powder

- 1/2 tsp. garlic powder

- One large egg

- 1/4 mug unsalted butter, melted and divided

- 1/2 mug shredded sharp Cheddar cheese one scallion, sliced

How to start

1. In a large pan, combine coconut flour, baking powder, and garlic powder.
2. Mix in egg, half of the melted butter, Cheddar cheese, and scallions. Put the batter into a 6" round baking pan. Put into the air fryer basket.
3. Adjust the temperature to 320°F and set the timer for 12 mins.
4. To serve, transfer from pan and allow to fully cool. Slice into four pieces and put the remaining melted butter over each.

PER SERVING

- Calories: 218
- Protein: 7.2grams Fiber: 3.4grams
- Net Carbohydrates : 3.4grams
- Fat: 16.9grams
- Sodium: 177 mg

- Carbohydrates: 6.8grams

- sugar: 2.1grams

51. Radish Chips

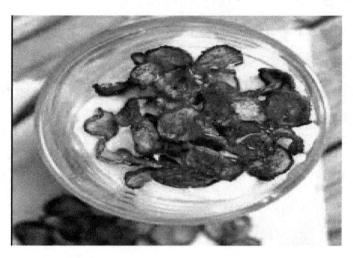

Hands on Time: 10 mins | Cook Time: 5 mins | Serving 4

Things We Need

- Two mugs water
- 1 pound radishes
- 1/4 tsp. onion powder
- 1/4 tsp. paprika
- 1/2 tsp. garlic powder
- 2 tbsp. coconut oil, melted

How to start

1. Put water in a medium pan and bring to a boil on the stovetop.

2. Transfer the top and bottom from each radish, and then use a mandolin to slice each radish thin and uniformly. You may also use the slicing blade in the food processor for this step.

3. Put the radish slices into the boiling water for 5 mins or until translucent. Transfer them from the water and put them into a clean kitchen towel to absorb excess moisture.

4. Toss the radish chips in a large pan with remaining ingredients until fully coated in oil and seasoning.

5. Place radish chips into it.

6. Set the temperature to 320°F and set the timer for 5 mins.

7. Shake the basket two or three times during the cooking time.

8. Serve warm.

PER SERVING

- Calories: 77
- Protein: 0.8 grams
- Fiber: 8 grams
- Net Carbohydrates : 2.2grams

- Fat: 6.5 grams
- Sodium: 40 mg
- Carbohydrates: 4.0grams
- sugar: 2.0 grams

52. Flatbread

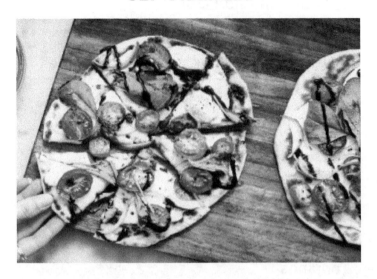

Hands on Time: 5 mins | Cook Time: 7 mins | Serving 2

Ingredients

- Peanut Sauce
- 2 tbsp. Rice Wine Vinegar
- 4 tbsp. Soy Sauce
- 4 tbsp. Reduced Sugar Ketchup
- 4 tbsp. Coconut Oil
- 1 tsp. Fish Sauce
- Juice of 1/2 Lime
- Pizza Base
- 2 cups Mozzarella Cheese (~8 oz.)

- 3/4 cup Almond Flour
- 1 tbsp. Psyllium Husk Powder
- 3 tbsp. Cream Cheese (~1.5 oz.)
- 1 large Egg
- 1/2 tsp. Onion Powder
- 1/2 tsp. Garlic Powder
- 1/2 tsp. Ginger
- 1/2 tsp. Salt
- 1/2 tsp. Pepper
- Toppings
- 2 Chicken Thighs
- 3 oz. Mung Bean Sprouts
- 6 oz. Mozzarella Cheese
- 2 medium Green Onions
- 1 1/2 oz. Shredded Carrot
- 2 tbsp. Peanuts

Instructions

1. One mug shredded mozzarella cheese 1/4 mug blanched finely ground almond flour 1-ounce full-Fat cream cheese, softened.

2. In a large microwave-safe pan, melt mozzarella in the microwave for 30 seconds. Mix in almond flour until smooth, and then add cream cheese.

Continue mixing until dough forms, gently kneading it with wet hands if necessary.

3. Divide the dough into two pieces and roll out to 1/4" thickness between two pieces of parchment. Cut another piece of parchment to fit your air fryer basket.

4. Put a piece of flatbread onto your parchment and into the air fryer, working in two batches if needed.

5. Set the temperature to 320°F and set the timer for 7 mins.

6. Halfway through the cooking time, flip the flatbread. Serve warm.

PER SERVING

- Calories: 296
- Protein: 16.3grams
- Fiber: 5 grams
- Net Carbohydrates : 3.3grams
- Fat: 22.6grams
- Sodium: 402 mg

- Carbohydrates: 4.8grams

- sugar: 5 grams

Conclusion

That fries is a little bit of an avalanche, a bitch, and an ace! Release to date, a Power Air Fryer, a cleaning tank is a simple pair. It may indeed be tough to clean the sea, and it will help us. Déanta a fírinne, which has been used to create the same philosophy and its use, is widespread, and this is again the case: BACON IS LIFE

CPSIA information can be obtained
at www.ICGtesting.com
Printed in the USA
LVHW080034280421
685734LV00008B/238